The Pill Popping Syndrome

Getting Rid of the Habit of Eating Unnecessary Pills/Drugs

Dueep Jyot Singh

Healthy Living Series

Mendon Cottage Books

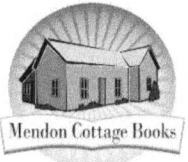

JD-Biz Publishing

Download Free Books!

http://MendonCottageBooks.com

Our books are available at

1. Amazon.com
2. Barnes and Noble
3. Itunes
4. Kobo
5. Smashwords
6. Google Play Books

Download Free Books!

http://MendonCottageBooks.com

Table of Contents

Introduction

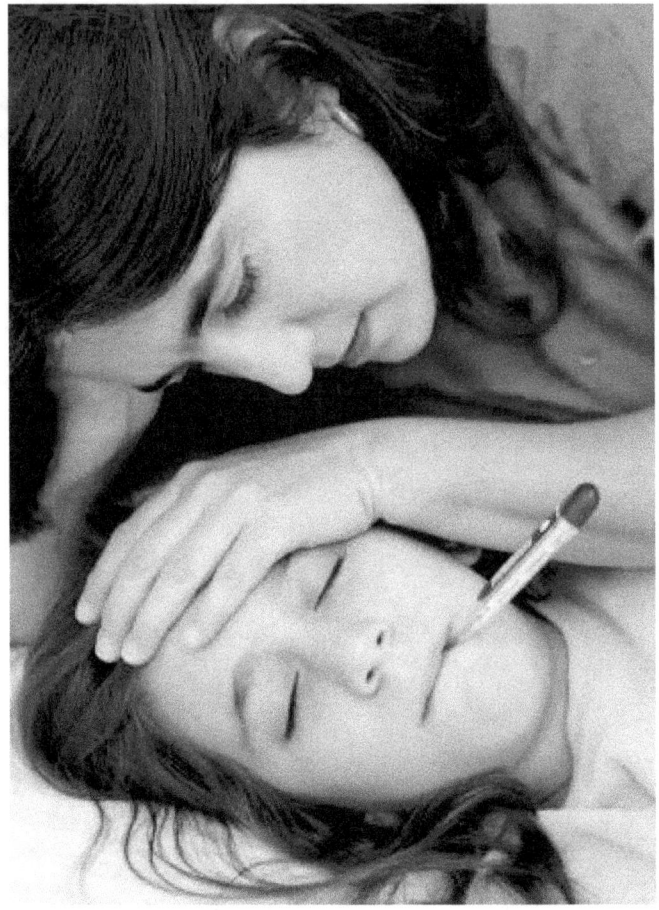

Apart from pills, how many times have you given your children syrups, medicines, prescription drugs, and antibiotics today?

A number of people out there are going to object to the use of the word/medical term "syndrome," associated with pill popping. Because according to them, they being purists, a syndrome is an association of symptoms, which characterize a particular ailment or condition, or a number of symptoms which are going to occur together in order to show the manifestation of an ailment.

Well, this book is going to tell you all about how you may think that a number of associated symptoms have caused you to suffer from some ailment, and the result is that you are going to start popping pills in order to alleviate those symptoms!

This book is going to tell you how you can recognize such a particular ailment/syndrome in yourself, try to wean yourself away from pills, and get back to the natural way of healing yourself of small disorders.

Also, you are going to get some information on possibly when and why pills began to become an important part of your normal day to day routine, and your lifestyle. So while you are reading this book, if you find yourself reaching for your pillbox, do not take that pill unless it is absolutely necessary and continue learning some interesting facts about the pills being taken by you every day.

Can you believe that 2.3 billion prescription drugs are prescribed to Americans alone, annually? That means 49% of you are taking at least one prescription drug, everyday, 22% are taking two or more drugs, and *11% are taking more than five prescription drugs every day.*

And this is in America alone. You can multiply this by whichever number you want, and get the world statistics.

Remember that there are some chronic diseases, especially those which are being monitored by a physician which need a daily dose of pills and drugs, in order to keep you alive. But 99% of the time, most of the pills that you take can be considered placebos or have been given to you by a doctor just because he needs to prescribe some medicines to you.

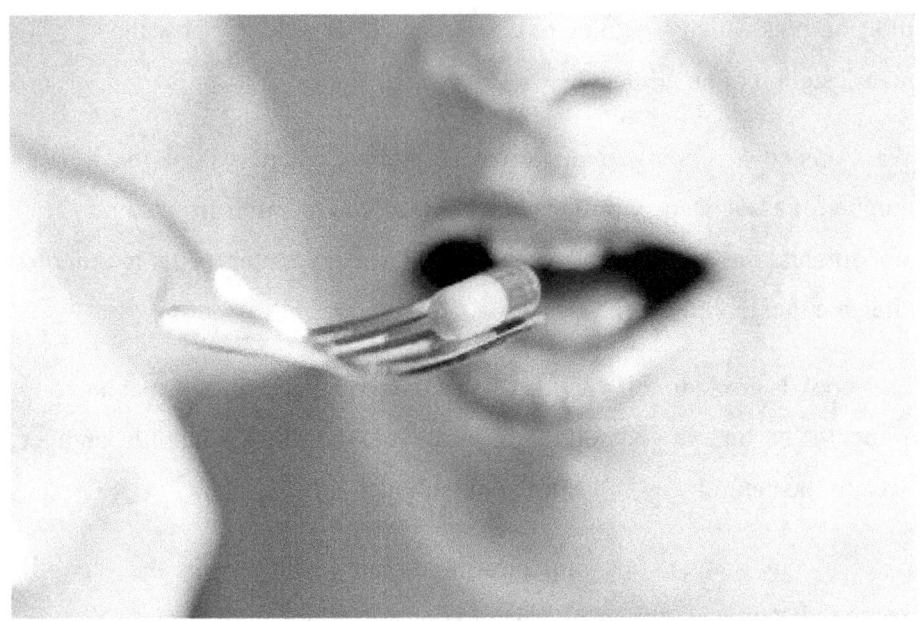

Are you eating pills as a substitute to healthy natural meals? Are you getting your nutrition from chemical-based vitamins and minerals and skipping meals? Is lunch and dinner just a number of drugs and medicines and supplements prescribed to you by your doctor?

On many occasions, many of these medicines are absolutely not necessary and are just placebos. So it is possible that a number of medicines which you are taking are given to you just to assure you that you are taking something in order to cure yourself. And this is where we come to the role of ancient medicine and placebos in our lives.

But before that, you would need to know the symptoms of a person suffering from a pill popping syndrome.

Pill Popping Syndrome – Symptoms

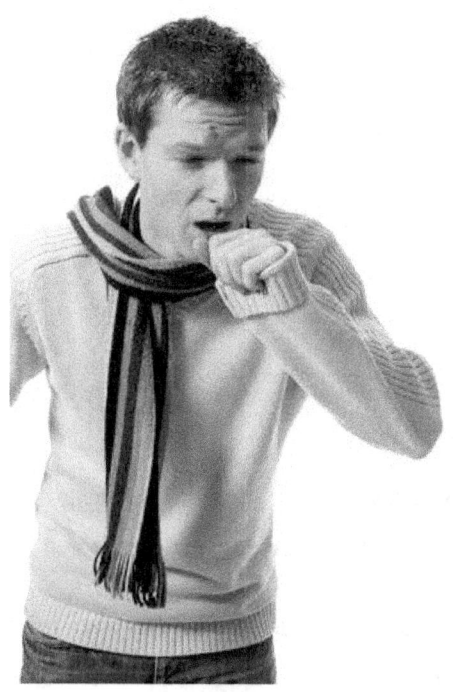

Oh Boy… This could be bronchitis, asthma, chest infections, throat infections, or any other serious chronic ailment. It could be an allergy or some rare disease. I need to take lots of pills in order to cure those infections and also to prevent any other sort of ailment from occurring.

Ignorance is bliss works both ways. Sometimes you may not know about a thing, and you do not worry about it. On the other hand, too much knowledge can also create too much confusion. Thanks to the large amount of knowledge available at our fingertips, we are our own doctors now. And naturally, this gives rise to more cases of hypochondriac behavior than anybody could guess. And that is why the pill popping syndrome is so much en vogue.

Most of us are suffering from this syndrome and addiction, but we do not know the symptoms.

Look at all the symptoms or any combination of one or two more of the symptoms? –

Are you suffering from

- Stress, strain and tension?

- Depression?

- Worry about the state of your health?

- Fear that if you do not take these pills, it is going to have an immediate overnight adverse affect on the state of your health?

- Start feeling jittery and nervous, if you have missed out on any dose of the pills prescribed to you by your doctor?

- Feel stressed-out, because your budget does not include enough money and funds in order to buy the monthly quota of prescribed drugs and pills for the full family?

I am sorry to say, my friend, that most of us are suffering from this syndrome. That is because we have been conditioned through our environment, media, doctors, healthcare workers, and corporate pharmaceutical brand names in such a manner since childhood itself that we are hundred percent terrified of not taking our daily dose of medicines.

And believe it or not, in 99% of the cases, it is not necessary for us to take these medicines, but thanks to the effect of these drugs on our natural bio – physiological and chemical makeup, which has been affected through this drug dependency, we immediately get stressed out because "Where Is My

Medicine? I Cannot Function without It. I Cannot Think Straight. Can't You See My Hand. It Is Shaking. I Just Need My Pills, to Get Back to Normal."

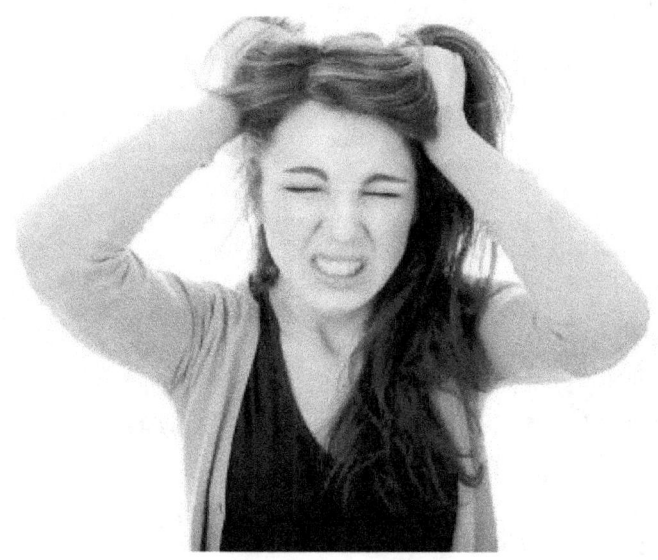

I need my pills, where are my pills, I have to have my pills, where are my pills, I should have already eaten them by now, where are my pills?

Incidentally, this was something I saw in one of my colleagues, to my great astonishment. She had been a perfectly normal healthy human being, until one of her doctors persuaded her that she was suffering from a number of ailments. *And after that, 60% of her monthly paycheck went in the buying of the medicines prescribed by her doctor.*

According to him, she was suffering from potential heart problems, potential high blood pressure, potential hypertension, potential immunodeficiency illnesses, and to prevent all of them from occurring, she had to take these medicines.

Do you notice that dangerous term, potential? Doctors and medical experts also tell their patients – "there is a possibility of…," "you may be genetically prone to…," "there is a chance that you may suffer from…," "you may need to undergo these tests in order to rule out the chances of…," And such other allied terms.

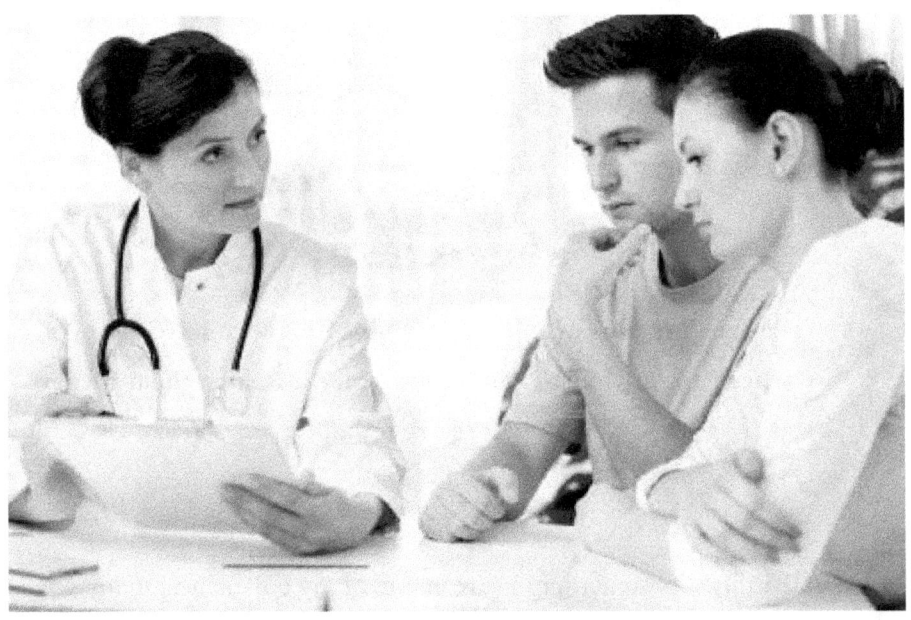

You cannot blame them, 5,000 years ago, mankind was undergoing the same psychological fright treatment from priests, – who would pray for your well-being on the payment of silver and gold, they were charlatans, quacks, swindlers, frauds, imposters, and fakes.

And because man is conditioned to believe the very worst, he fell into the hands of those very clever people, all those millenniums ago. Even though most of those medicines were just placebos.

Placebos

Believe it or not, for millenniums, physicians have been giving pills, medicines, syrups, decoctions, medical preparations, lotions, and potions to their patients just for psychological effect, and which may auto suggest the patient into curing himself. These have absolutely nothing to do with natural remedies and medicines.

These are known as placebos and are made up of ordinary items like powdered sugar, powdered herbs, and anything which is not going to do any sort of harm to your system. And you are going to take this medicine, thinking it to be effective in order to cure your ailment. And 99% of the time, it is going to be cured.

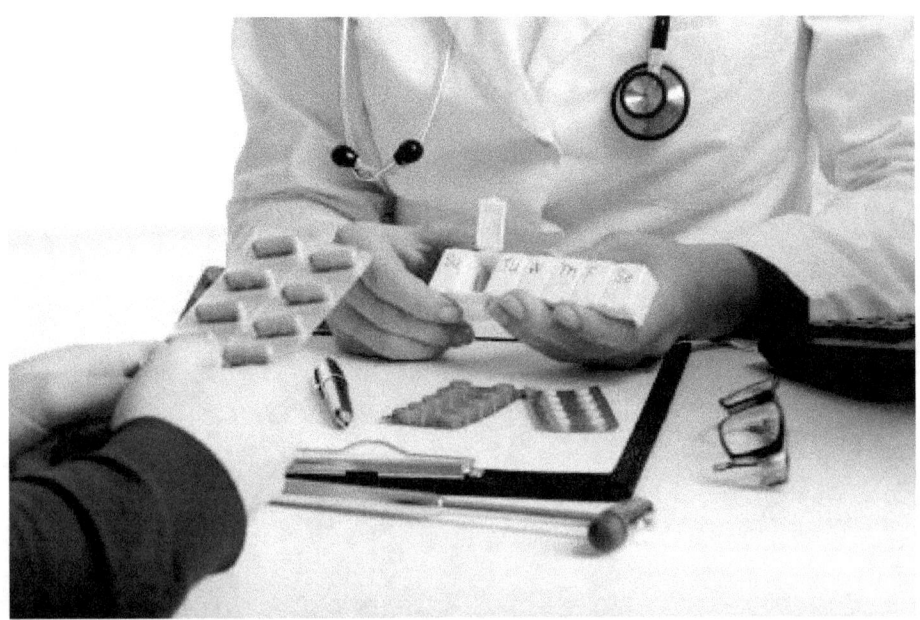

Let me tell you a 600-year-old story as said in Persian mythology. In the time of caliphs, there was a very well known physician, who was well known throughout the land for finding the cure for all of your ills. One day he was called in by the caliph, who seemed to have some unknown malady, which made him feel lethargic, unenergetic, bored, tired, listless, and thus he supposed himself ill.

The physician immediately checked the caliph's pulse and then made some pensive Hmmmmmm noises which pleased the caliph greatly. He seemed to be suffering from some really serious ailment, if one went by the thoughtful mien of the physician.

And then the physician spoke – "Oh great Caliph, you have a really rare disease. The treatment is going to be expensive. I may have to use some powdered pearls. You will have to take three doses every day. Apart from this, you are going to run around the palace ground, once, every morning, in the fresh air saying, "Get thee, away from me, oh wicked ailment, in the name of Allah." And as you take God's name, you are going to see this ailment going away from you, because evil things cannot stay where God's name is taken. But you need to take that medicine regularly for three months.

Within one week, the caliph began to feel much better. Within one week. He found himself really energetic. Within three months, he considered himself completely cured.

He called the physician in, and took off a necklace of valuable stones from around his neck, and put it around the neck of the physician. And then he praised him for his medicine. The treatment was expensive but it was worth it.

The physician immediately told him the way in which he could keep that particular ailment away for the rest of his life, and requested him to call him, whenever he was needed, ever again.

Later on the physician's wife told her husband what could have happened if the Caliph knew that he was being fed little packages of powdered sugar and for which the Caliph was paying such a high price?

The wise physician smiled and said, "Know this, oh lady of the house, that he is the Caliph. If he was not given a really rare and expensive medicine which was exotic, and full of wonderful ingredients bought at a very high price, he would still be leading an idle life, without any exercise and imagining himself to be sick. I have now put him on a regime of keeping busy throughout the day in physical activities, and walking among the poor in order to find what ails them. And being the Caliph, it is his job to alleviate their suffering, in order to prevent his suffering from coming back. This is going to keep him mentally busy too and occupied throughout the day. He is not going to have any time to be idle thinking up ailments or deciding that he is sick."

We loved this story told to us when we were children by our father. And throughout our childhood, whenever we thought that we were ill or headachy, he used to tell us – "you want some powdered pearls?" And we used to giggle.

We were then immediately turned out into the garden to do some constructive work like digging, or just jumping about in the fresh air.

Naturally, we never ate any medicines, when we were children. That was because we were not taught the medicine culture. Fresh air, good food, plenty of exercise, and absolutely no pandering to any ailments meant that even when we grew up there was absolutely no question of our eating any medicines, going to hospitals, or taking any pills ever.

How many human beings all over the world can assert this freedom from pills, especially if they are living in well developed countries?

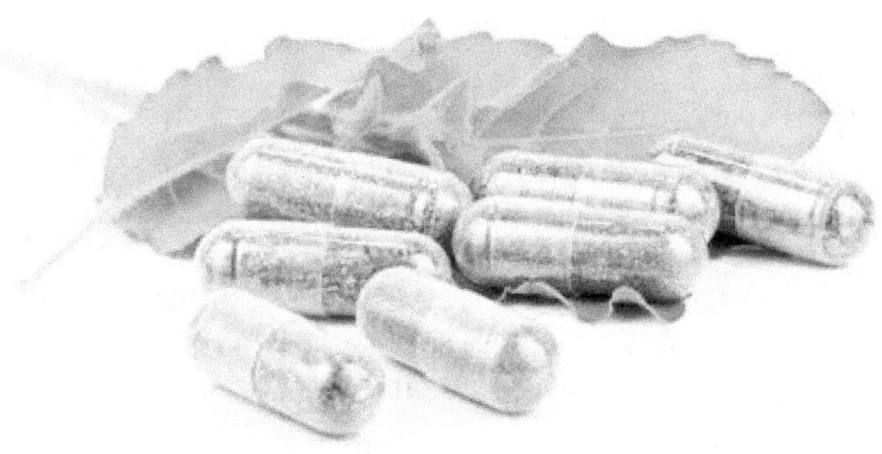

Well, my father has something to say about this, according to his experience in America. If we go by the time perspective, especially in America, vitamins and pills were given to soldiers and officers during the Second World War, in order to prevent any sort of nutritional or mineral deficiency due to a lack of proper food. These vitamins and supplements were prescribed by their Army doctors.

But the wholesale eating of vitamins, medicines, drugs, and supplements was not a normal thing in late 1959, which was when my father was a part of a 100 man strong team of professional engineers, invited from different parts of the World, by the American government to undergo steel training programs in reputed engineering colleges all over America.

He was a member of the third batch, and he recounts that the members of the first batch were given such huge allowances that they began saving up the money, instead of spending it on food and drink! Within two years, they had enough money with which they could buy plenty of expensive things like refrigerators, cooker ranges, and other such items to take back home, on payments of cash!

By the time, the third batch was ready to come to America, the American government and sponsors had learned a bit of financial good sense. The daily/monthly allowances were reduced to just enough on which the trainees could survive, throughout the day/month!

And when they said that the food and the drink was expensive, they were given handfuls of *pills and supplements.* This was supposed to be compensation enough for any nutritional deprivation, which would occur through loss of meals or not being able to eat a well-balanced and nutritional diet, just because one could not afford to do so!

Incidentally, about this time, the Pres. Eisenhower [1] administration was confronted with a Nationwide Steel Workers strike. That is when doctors

---

[1] I, in very admiring tones – "you mean you and your fellow batch mates were invited to the White House and met Pres. Eisenhower? Did you eat anything there?" Father's reply – "I am not quite sure I remember what I ate, but it was healthy, tasty and natural home-cooked food. If it was anything else, I would have noted it." I can

began to worry about the health of the workers, because if they did not work, they did not earn. And that means they would compromise on their meals, cutting out on food items just because they could not afford to buy them. And that meant the overall general quality of their health would suffer.

And that is when doctors started prescribing pills, nutritional supplements, vitamins, and minerals in a pill form to the workers, to compensate for any nutritional deficiency brought about through malnutrition and starvation.

And so healthcare centers were told to hand out pills, vitamins, minerals, and other chemical-based nutritional supplements in handfuls, to the workers and their families, so that they could keep healthy.

Notice this? The idea was being promulgated subconsciously that you do not need to eat healthy food when you can make do with vitamins and other supplements given to you by your doctors and healthcare workers, in the form of pills and supplements.

And so, in the 1960s, pharmaceutical companies, learned that this was a good way in which they could sell lots and lots of vitamins, minerals, and nutritional supplements to everyone in America, – they had already seen the way in which steelworkers and other professional people doing physical

---

well believe that, because he is a gourmand and enjoys his food in whichever country he finds himself in.

So, at that time, Pres. Eisenhower ["Gen. Eisenhower", according to Dad] insisted on a natural, healthy, nourishing diet in the White House because he had been brought up on it. So what happened, to American eating habits and lifestyles since then? Read on…

labor were being encouraged by government agencies and medical agencies to take these pills and supplements.

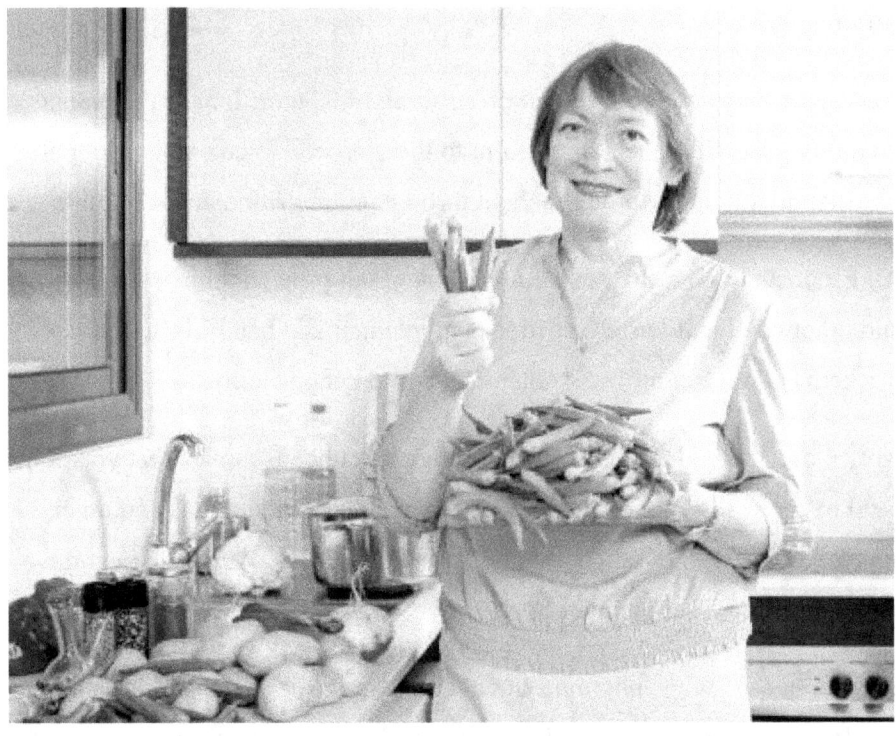

There is absolutely no way in the World in which any pill, medicine, nutritional supplement, or anything manufactured in labs can take the place of the natural nutrients supplied to you through natural, healthy, organic fresh food.

And so you can understand how the people of that generation began to eat these pills in handfuls. What they did not know was that this was the beginning of the end and the slow erosion of natural good health, which was their genetic inheritance and which they had kept intact, through the eating of available nourishing and nutritional food.

Incidentally, when my father came back, he was so healthy because his stay in America, eating a high protein diet, plenty of nutritional food, fruit, vegetables, milk, and absolutely no pills and supplements – even though he was given them by the handful by his sponsors – that even today, he persists on that same lifestyle.

And he is astonished to hear that in the last 60 years or more, Americans who were supposed to be one of the healthiest people on earth, at that time due to their good and balanced diets are now more interested in ruining their health, and replacing good natural honest-to-goodness food and meals with pills?

Now, let us come to the 70s. This was the time when the brainwashing idea of you need to have so many medicines to eat in order to keep healthy, had begun to affect people globally.

And these included doctors!

Somewhere around '76, one of my father's men was injured in an accident and taken to the base hospital. After checking on the well-being of the patient, my father went in to see the doctor in charge, Dr. M.[2] and was astonished to see the doctor say, "just a moment, sir," and then in front of

---

[2] Dr. M and I had a running feud – both of us "disliked" each other cordially. I considered him quite a dumbbell and stupid adult, and he kept wondering how I managed to keep alive, being brought in to the hospital, every third day, due to some injury or the other. And making lots of work for him. He told me so point-blank. And any medicines, he gave me I just threw out of the window, because I did not trust him!

dad, he took out a number of pills – dad says that they may have been anywhere between 8 to 14 – asked the nearest hospital attendant to give him a glass full of water, and gulped them down.

Father immediately asked him whether it was necessary for a doctor to eat so many medicines, and Dr. M said that they were vitamins, supplements, blood thinners, stress relievers, and *other medicines he had prescribed to himself.* That is when our feud started, because I was rude and tactless and said very loudly that only monkeys eat so many medicines in fistfuls.[3]

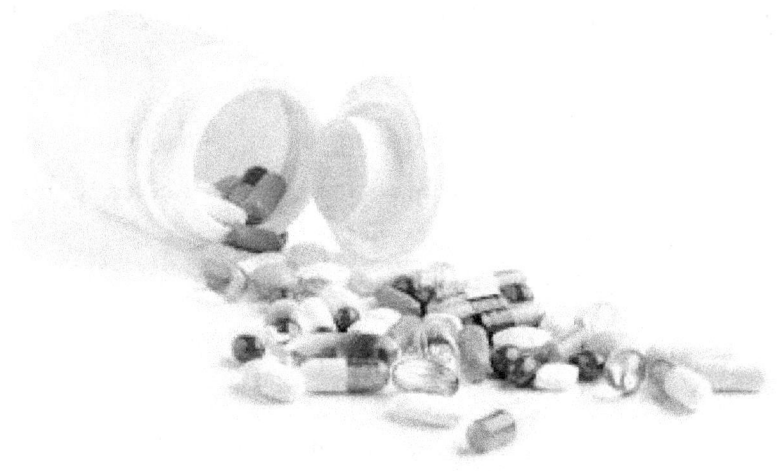

---

[3] Dr. Mankar was immediately dubbed Dr. Monkey and he never forgave me for that, especially due to his unfortunate surname. I was a spoiled brat. I was also rude, nasty, obnoxious, and those were just some of my good qualities, according to Dr. M. According to him, I would have been well improved by a timely drowning at birth! On the other hand, his Senior, Colonel S. and I were very good friends, because he never talked down to me or acted facetious or arch. Children do not like that sort of superior patronizing behavior ever on the part of adults.

It was when I grew up and began to get interested in the medical field and science as a future career, that I began to see just how much the pharmaceutical companies all over the world had had a stronghold on the medical profession.

Doctors and the Hippocratic Oath

The original Hippocratic oath spoken in Greek called upon a number of Gods to help in the healing of mankind. Hippocrates lived in the fifth century, this oath was written sometimes later, as a moral guide ruling the ethical and professional behavior of doctors down the ages.

It is one of the most important documents in human history, taking into view the social, economic, traditional, cultural, scientific, and other changes undergone by humankind and society down the ages.

Here is a part of the original Greek oath,

I will apply dietetic measures for the benefit of the sick according to my ability and judgment; I will keep them from harm and injustice.

I will neither give a deadly drug to anybody who asked for it, nor will I make a suggestion to this effect. Similarly I will not give to a woman an abortive remedy. In purity and holiness I will guard my life and my art.

Times have changed, but all time moral values and ethics should still hold. Especially when it is the responsibility of the doctor to give the patient proper knowledge of a right diet and nonprescription of a harmful drug – we are using the term deadly drug here in its broadest sense.

Doctors were encouraged to prescribe a large number of drugs and medicines to their patients, and they still are doing that, all over the world, without even bothering about the harmful results and side effects of such an administration.

So these patients are not patients at all. They are just guinea pigs being fed drugs which have been banned in other parts of the World, but have been sent to developing countries and third World countries by multibillion-dollar pharmaceutical companies who want to keep up their profits without counting the cost to human rights and life.

Once, when I asked one of my doctor friends, why she was prescribing a medicine to a patient, of which the side effect was well known, – which had been banned in Europe, UK, and in America but was easily available in Africa, Asia, and other parts of the World – and would give rise to another set of problems, she just shrugged her shoulders and said that the medical samples were being given to her free by pharmaceutical company representatives, *so she was just passing them on to her patients.*

And these are the doctors who speak the Hippocratic Oath.

http://guides.library.jhu.edu/c.php?g=202502&p=1335759

You can read this oath in its modern entirety here. How many of the doctors that you know today are following it? When I told her that she was following the Hypocritical Oath, she gave me a look of How Glad I Am That You Did Not Join Medical College, along with the Rest of Us, You Pain in the Neck Do-Gooder, and told me to scoot because she was busy.

Believe it or not, friends, I am not a scaremongering person, just writing about controversial things in order to boost up my sales, but I am telling you the truth. I have been a hospital administrator. I have seen a number of these drugs being given by the bag full to the doctors on my panel, for the treatment of a number of diseases, in the number of fields including urology, cardiology, gynecology, pediatrics, geriatrics, and neurosurgery.

And I have seen a number of doctors saying that these medicines, according to medical journals, were not safe to be administered and they had been banned in a number of countries. And they could take the medicines back.

And once I heard one of these pharmaceutical company representatives telling the doctor Point blank – "Why should you bother, Doctor? If the patient improves, he is proof that the medicine works. If he does not improve, you can just say that the medicine was all right, but the patient's condition was such that even this particular medicine could not help."

So, friends, human beings, this should show you that you are not considered to be living, breathing human beings in the scheme of a multibillion-dollar pharmaceutical and medical corporate industry. You are just guinea pigs.

And that is why you are going to be persuaded to take a number of medicines which are certain to debilitate your natural immune system and incapacitate your body's natural capacity of healing itself.

So start thinking for yourself and decide to change your lifestyle right now.

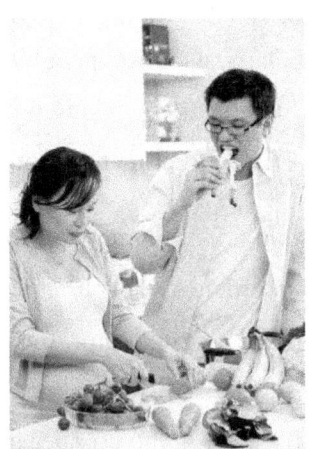

A healthy new generation all over the world can occur only when parents are sensible about their diet, nutrition, nourishment, and do not contaminate natural nutrients with unessential supplements and pills, prescribed, suggested, advised, or just told to them by all and sundry.

Your body is not a depository of a chemical lab. It is a basically healthy natural power factory which can only keep healthy, as long as you do not adulterate your food with chemical-based supplements sold by pharmaceutical companies or change the basic natural genetic and bio-physiological makeup of your body and perhaps your genes with lots of prescription drugs.

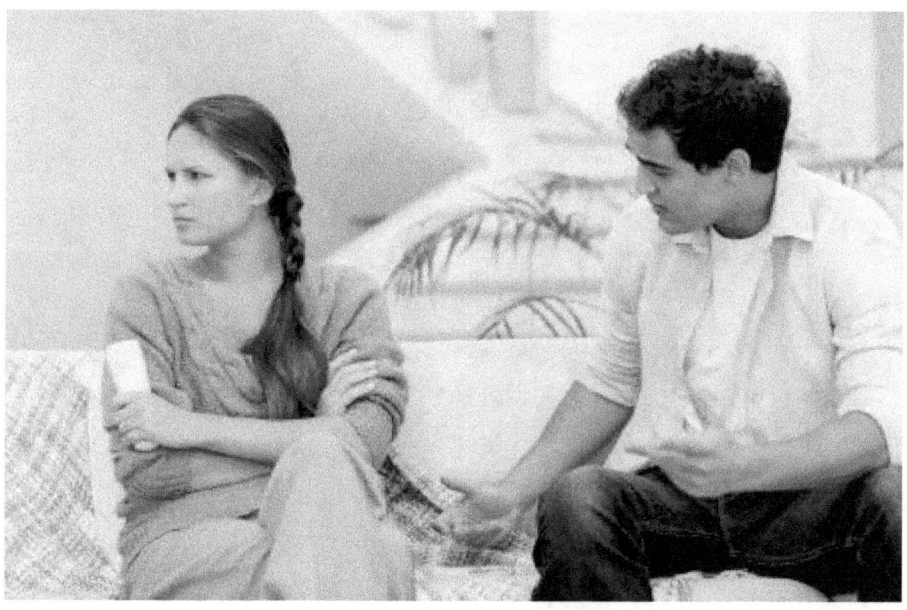

Why are you getting angry with me? I just asked you to ask your doctor to change your medicine, because the side effect of the last medicine, that he prescribed to you was loss of concentration and change in behavior. And then he prescribed another medicine to you to counteract that side effect, which had another side effect – loss of temper and impatience. What is my fault here?

Weaning Yourself Away from Pills

This is going to be extremely difficult, especially if you have been conditioned since childhood to believe that your existence depends on these medicines.

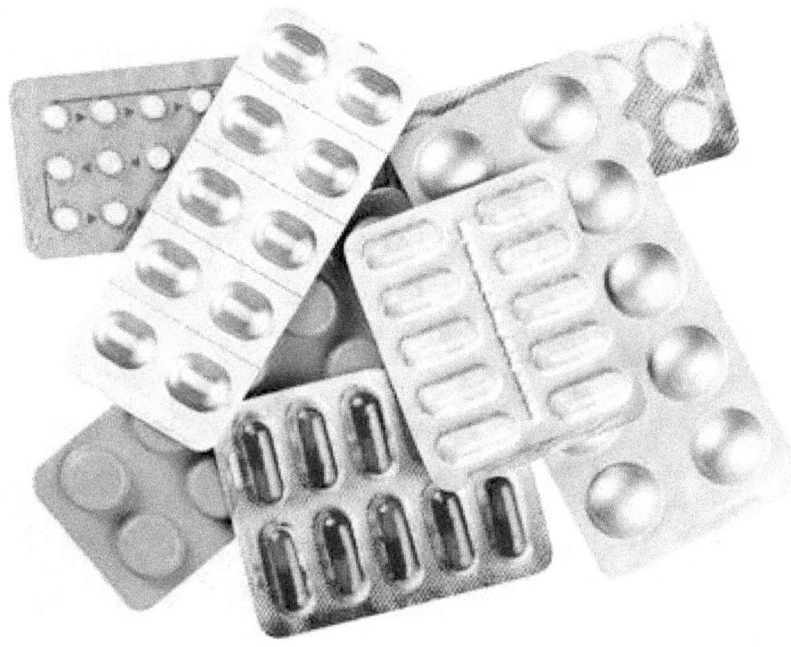

That does not mean that I am denigrating some of the miracles done by dedicated doctors. They are the ones who believe in the true meaning of being a doctor in its full form. They are the ones – including Dr. M and Col. S – who kept me alive throughout my accident-prone childhood and youth! They are the doctors who brought me back from the dead three times in my life, because they just would not give up. And those are the doctors. I revere and respect.

My target are all those doctors, who could not care less about the well-being of their patients. Their job is to make money.

Let me tell you about the story of a little girl I know who was born with a heart condition. At the age of eight, the doctors felt that she was strong enough to undergo an operation, and the operation was successful. When she came out of the operating theater, her first words were "Where is the pain? And did all human beings go through this pain from childhood itself?"

One can only applaud the skill of the doctors, and when her doctor asked her why she was asking this question, she said that ever since she was a baby, she walked hand-in-hand with pain. And she thought that every human being went through that same purgatory until the age of eight.

Some very busy doctor had not bothered to tell her that she was suffering from a heart condition since birth. He just gave her medicines in order to stabilize her condition. He did not bother about her emotional and mental needs, he was just bothered about keeping her alive and incidentally getting a hefty monthly payment for those medicines from her parents.

This child needed these medicines. But do you?

But here I am discussing how you can wean yourself away from pills and forget about the pill popping syndrome.

Look into your medicine cabinet. How many pills are there, which had been prescribed to you sometime or the other on your visits to doctors?

How many of these medical treatment courses have you gone through in their entirety?

How many thousands of dollars have you spent in medical treatments, going through expensive procedures for a number of ailments? In many cases, it may be necessary, especially when there is no other option. But in the other cases, was it necessary for you to go to the doctor?

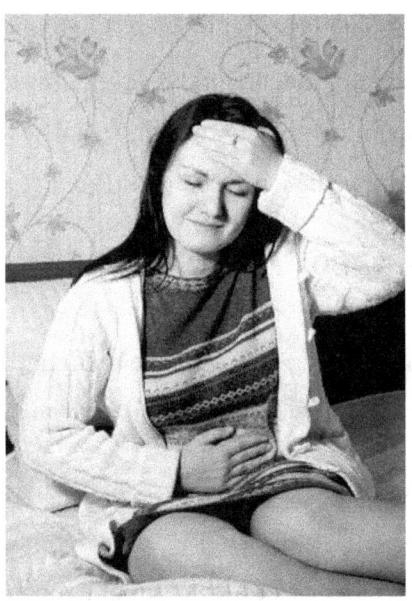

It looks like a tummy upset again. I will have to take that red pill, and that green and white pill and that yellow pill, oh and that blue pill and also that green liquid. I just hope that this problem goes away by tomorrow.

Notice, that this lady is so used to popping pills, which supposedly give her temporary relief, that she has begun prescribing her medicines for herself. It may not be a tummy upset. It may be something else. But she is so used to taking all those medicines that she is going to pop them down and hope for the best.

If it is something dangerous, there is absolutely no chance that it will have gone away by the next morning. And so she is going to take some more medicines in order to cure herself.

If she is fortunate and lucky, she may get cured. If she is unlucky, she is going to come down with another set of side effects and symptoms, which are going to be treated with another set of pills.

And so the circle is going to go on in a really vicious downward spiral, which is bad for your health, physical and mental, as well as emotional well-being and, naturally, also your purse.

How many of us are our own doctors out there? Sadly enough, a number of us resort to this last-ditch effort, because we have lost faith in the power of the medical profession to cure us, we do not trust them, or we find their medical treatment extremely expensive and beyond our means.

This is the reason why remember in the introduction, I told you that 49% of Americans are taking at least one prescription drug. More and more Americans are slowly and steadily trying to look for alternative medicine options which can help cure them permanently instead of temporarily.

And this of course has terrified the pharmaceutical companies. If their general public does not buy the medicines they are churning out, they need to try alternatives. This includes telling the general public that any sort of alternative medicine is harmful to them. Natural remedies are not beneficial, and alternative medicine processes, like Chinese, Indian, Korean, Japanese, and other ancient medicines are not to be trusted because believe it or not, here is one slogan said in the 60s, when speaking against other medicine alternatives – "his Is All Communist Propaganda and Is Not the American Way.

Today, they cannot say that this is all Communist propaganda. But they are still persisting on this is not the American way. So what is the American way? You should continue eating their expensive drugs and spoil your health? You should be so dependent on the pills they prescribed to you, because they said so and it is patriotic for you to listen to what they say?

Think for yourself my friend. Did you ever ask your doctor for any sort of alternative medicine and his first reaction was – "No no no, do not take that medicine. It is harmful, and it is going to kill you. My medicines are helping you, are not they? If you stop eating my medicines, I am not responsible for your future bad health. I stabilize your condition with my prescription medicines. And what are you thinking of doing, who gave you the idea of alternative medicines? Don't you know that those natural foodstuffs and diets are prescribed by quacks, but I am a qualified doctor."

All of this is being told to you with a stern look, so that you begin to feel that you are so disloyal, letting all his good work go to dust, just because you thought of trying out some other alternative remedy.

And so you continue eating those prescribed pills and paying those expensive bills.

So coming back to weaning yourself away from the pills, think of all those pills, which you have not eaten. Why did you stop eating them? Just because you decided not to go through the full course prescribed by your doctor.

Then look at all those pills on your table, which you may eat throughout the day. How many of them are vitamins and supplements? How many of them have been prescribed, because your doctor found some deficiency in you and told you to buy an expensive branded name?

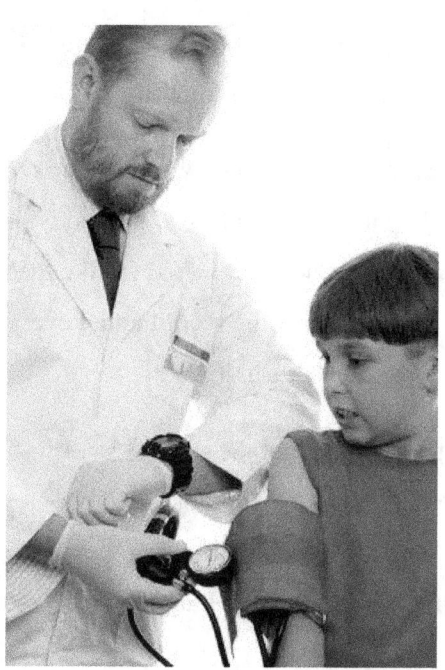

If this is a normal checkup, that is all well and good. But if this little boy has to go every week to get his treatment done for a disease, for which he is still being tested and drugs being prescribed to him, stop this shortening of his life immediately! Allow him to live a healthy, normal life, away from under the shadow of the stethoscope.

You have bought all these medicines, because like I said before, you are persuaded that you cannot do without them. You can do without them. So unless they are absolutely necessary to keep you alive, just get rid of them.

My grandmother was 84, at that time and I was visiting her, when I found a really distinguished looking gentleman as her guest, brought to her by one of her friends. This gentleman had managed to impress her greatly, with plenty of spiritual talk, and he was even more persuasive when he began to talk about one of the expensive medicines which he had just found out which were made up of natural mushroom extract. These mushrooms were found in mountainous areas in remote patches.

And that is why the medical supplement which he was talking to her about was very expensive. But it was going to stop her body organs from deteriorating due to old age. She would need to take these extracts and supplements for eight months, and he would come every month to give her her month's quota on payment, cash down.

She was just going to go in and get the cash, when I just said, "Grandma, just wait." He immediately gave me a look of "Now, now, then, young kids should be seen and not heard, especially when their elders are talking," and I said very respectfully, "Grandpa Sir,[4] I am so impressed with your mushroom extract."

He relaxed a little. This kid seemed to be a well brought up kid.

I continued, "That means you are going to give grandma this medicine for eight months and that is going to stop her natural aging process and stop her body from weakening any further? It is wonderful. What is the diet she is going to be taking along with that?"

"Oh, her normal diet, my child," said he beaming approvingly on me.

"That means after eight months, when she stops this medicine, she is going to be really healthy, with lots of energy and young and rejuvenated?"

---

[4] This is the respectful term with which elders are addressed in the East, to show that you revere their experience and white hair and age!

"Oh, no no no, the first eight months is only for steadying her body system, and stopping it from deterioration. The rest of her life, she is going to eat this medicine in order to keep young and to prevent her body from failing."

I just looked at my grandmother, who was looking at him open mouthed. I did not say anything except "Grandma, USD300. Every month. For the rest of your life!"

Grandma could not get rid of him fast enough. Though she never thanked me, because her friend was so horrified at this insult and disrespect shown to such a knowledgeable person, that she never spoke to grandma again.

Grandma died at the age of 95, 10 years ago, – she slipped in the bathroom and had a hemorrhage – and if that had not occurred, she would have been healthy, hearty, and all today, without any resort to expensive exotic mushroom extracts. And as she had warned everybody in her circle against buying that mushroom extract supplement, and using a major part of their army pensions in buying these expensive fads, is it a wonder that nobody came to our house in order to sell things to her, especially when I was around.

I asked such awkward questions.

And now let us come to another part of what happens when you go to a hospital.

This was about six years ago. December 17th, and I had fallen sick because of bad water because of a location change. Three days later, when my father found that I was incapable of eating anything except a piece of bread in three days, he decided to break his rule of never going to a hospital and consulted a doctor.

The moment he said that my daughter has not eaten anything except a piece of bread for the past three days, he was subjected to an *Oh yeah, do not exaggerate*, look by the doctor. This immediately put his back up. He was not used to his word not being believed.

When father told him my symptoms of high fever, joint pains, and continuous vomiting, the doctor immediately perked up and said, "It could be dengue. It could be hepatitis B. We have to find out. Should I send the ambulance? You say that she has been vomiting. That means she is suffering from dehydration. She has to be brought to the hospital immediately, for extensive medical testing. We will admit her immediately into the ICU."

My father ran from the doctor as fast as he could, while the doctor was still asking for his address! Within five days, I was all right, being fed on nourishing homemade chicken soup made by father and pieces of buttered bread.

He had just given me half a tablet of ibuprofen to bring the fever down, somewhere on the 19th. That is one over the counter drug, he keeps in his medicine cabinet just for emergencies. By the 22nd, I was back to normal, and ready for work, restored through chicken soup and getting back my strength through milk, fruit, eggs, boiled meat, and green vegetables and other healthy nourishing food.

What if father had been really scared by the doctor's terrifying tone and brought me to the hospital? I would have had to spend thousands of dollars on drugs, medical treatments, and procedures which would have prevented my natural immune system from curing my body naturally.

So like I said, think about it.

Start eating natural foods. Stop eating those pills. Stop worrying about the bad after effects which are going to occur if you stop using drugs and medicines which you take to keep yourself beautiful and youthful. Stop spending your life at the beck and call of medicines.

You may find yourself suffering from the symptoms given above, stress, tension, and strain, because you have been persuaded to think that you cannot do without these medicines.

Just imagine that you have been hit by hurricane Freya. Survival is your first priority. You could not manage to grab your pill bag, with all your vitamin supplements and other medicines.

And just imagine God forbid that you are now in circumstances where you have no access to any of these medical supplies including supplements. So how are you going to survive? By learning how to eat the food which is available to you, without access to processed foods and fast foods.

And you are going to find yourself healthier, because you have again come back to nature.

Think it over.

Conclusion

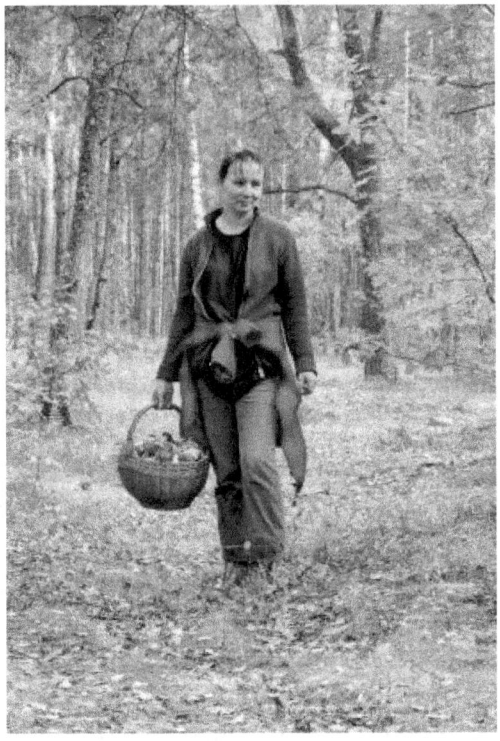

Fresh air and food, and a more natural way of living should be what you should aim for, as a future healthy lifestyle.

Now that you have come to the end of this book, do not ever be under the impression that all Americans, or even a majority of the people in developed countries out there are pill poppers. That is not so. My aunt Kathie is one of the healthiest Americans I know, and I have never seen her taking a pill. On the other hand, another aunt of mine, Cuckie, cannot do without three pills three times a day, in her little pillbox, and when I asked her what they were, she told me that they were her vitamin and mineral supplements, prescribed to her by her doctor in sunny LA.

She has been eating them for the last 51 years, ever since she first met that doctor who she trusts implicitly, but for him she is his human guinea pig. He tests out all his medicines on her. And then he tests out the medicines given to him to counteract the side effects of the previous prescriptions.

And she thinks that he is just wonderful. And her youth, good health, and beauty[5] are due to his medicines.

I did not tell her that she is managing to survive, because she walks 10 – 15 miles every day and eats lots of fruit and vegetables and never diets, even though her system has been totally poisoned by these drugs.

But then, I am not here to persuade you to go against your doctor's wishes, if you think he is just wonderful.

However, try your best to stop eating all those useless medicines, most of which you do not need. Try changing your lifestyle and getting out more into the air.

Remember, the future state of your health is in your hands. If you hate the thought of changing your diet and incorporating more fruit and vegetables into it, because you are not used to eating them, look online.

There are so many interesting sites, where you can try out fruit and vegetable recipes from all over the World, and make them into salads, chutneys, dips, spreads, or any other dishes which are anything but bland, bland, bland.

So flourish, Live Long and Prosper!

---

[5] No comment.

Author Bio

Dueep Jyot Singh is a Management and IT Professional who managed to gather Postgraduate qualifications in Management and English and Degrees in Science, French and Education while pursuing different enjoyable career options like being an hospital administrator, IT,SEO and HRD Database Manager/ trainer, movie , radio and TV scriptwriter, theatre artiste and public speaker, lecturer in French, Marketing and Advertising, ex-Editor of Hearts On Fire (now known as Solstice) Books Missouri USA, advice columnist and cartoonist, publisher and Aviation School trainer, ex-moderator on Medico.in, banker, student councilor ,travelogue writer … among other things!

One fine morning, she decided that she had enough of killing herself by Degrees and went back to her first love -- writing. It's more enjoyable! She already has 48 published academic and 14 fiction- in- different- genre books under her belt.

When she is not designing websites or making Graphic design illustrations for clients , she is browsing through old bookshops hunting for treasures, of which she has an enviable collection – including R.L. Stevenson, O.Henry, Dornford Yates, Maurice Walsh, De Maupassant, Victor Hugo, Sapper, C.N. Williamson, "Bartimeus" and the crown of her collection- Dickens "The Old Curiosity Shop," and "Martin Chuzzlewit" and so on… Just call her "Renaissance Woman" - collecting herbal remedies, acting like Universal Helping Hand/Agony Aunt, or escaping to her dear mountains for a bit of exploring, collecting herbs and plants, and trekking.

Check out some of the other JD-Biz Publishing books

Gardening Series on Amazon

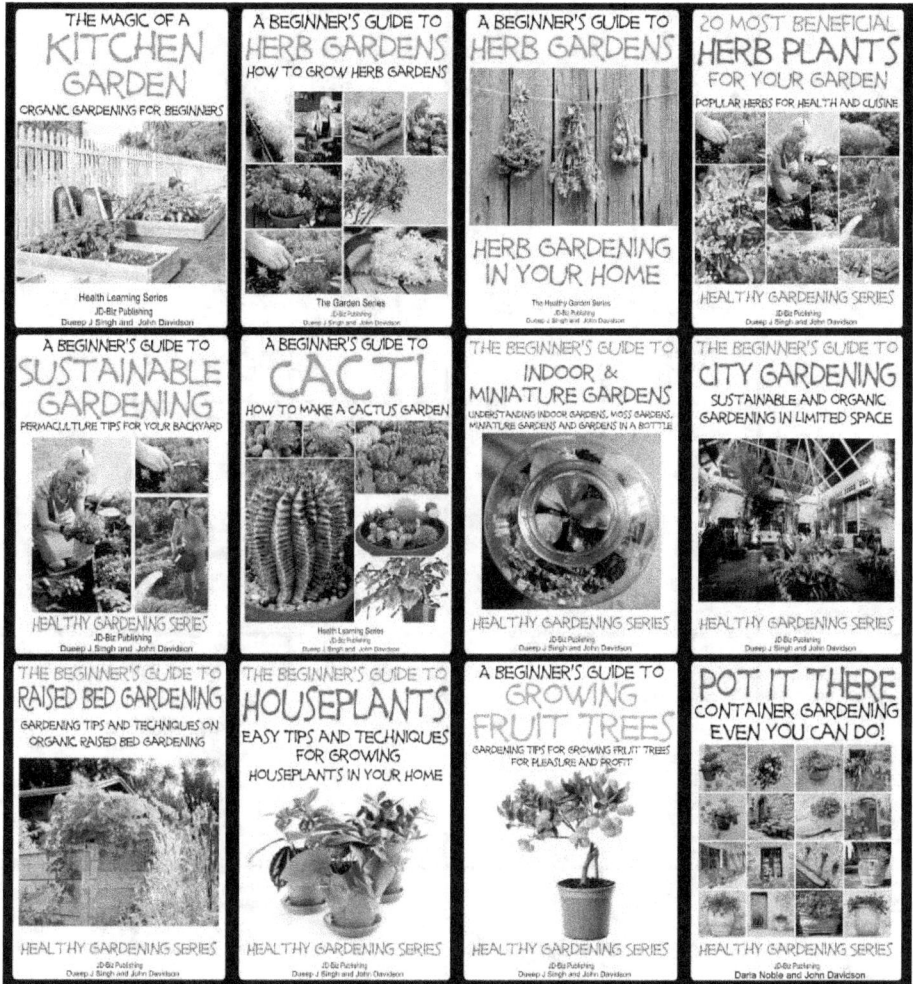

Download Free Books!

http://MendonCottageBooks.com

Health Learning Series

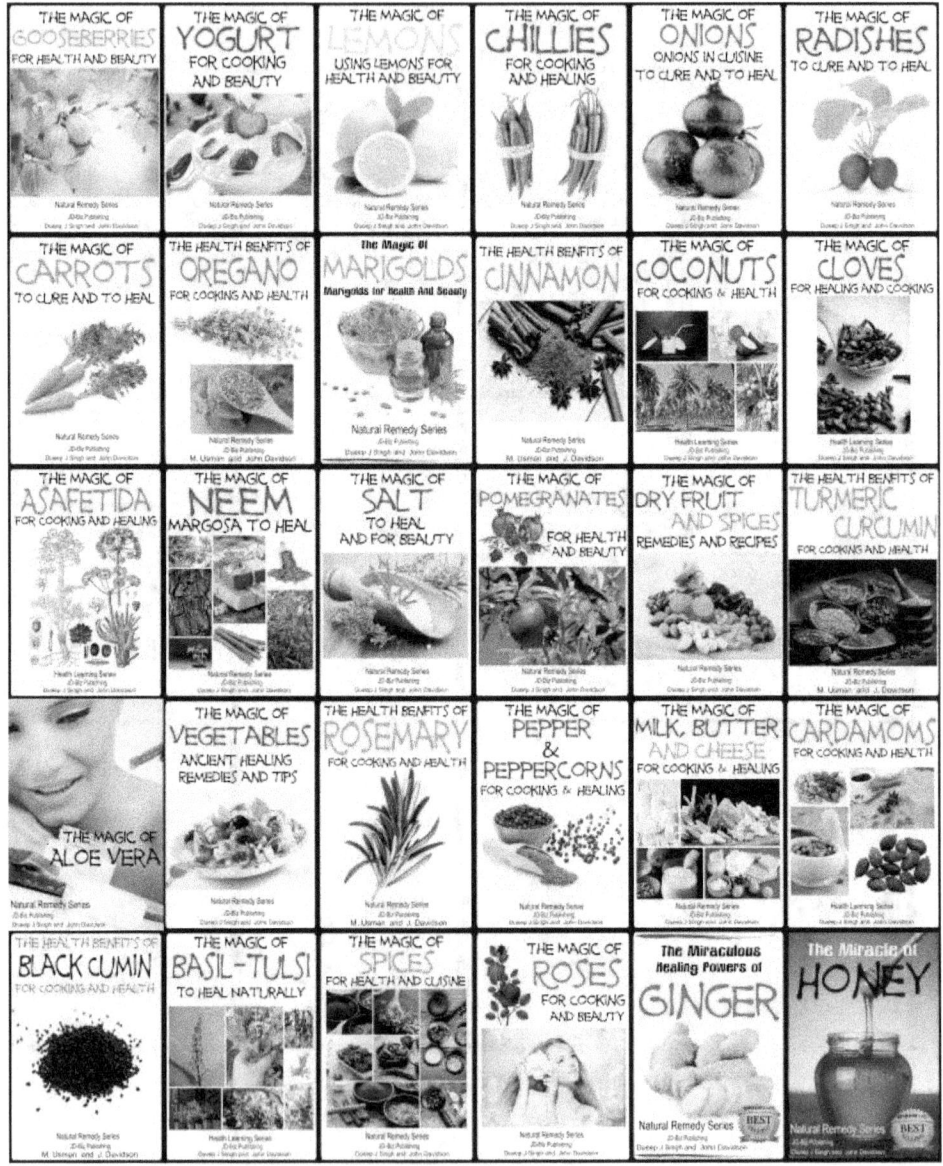

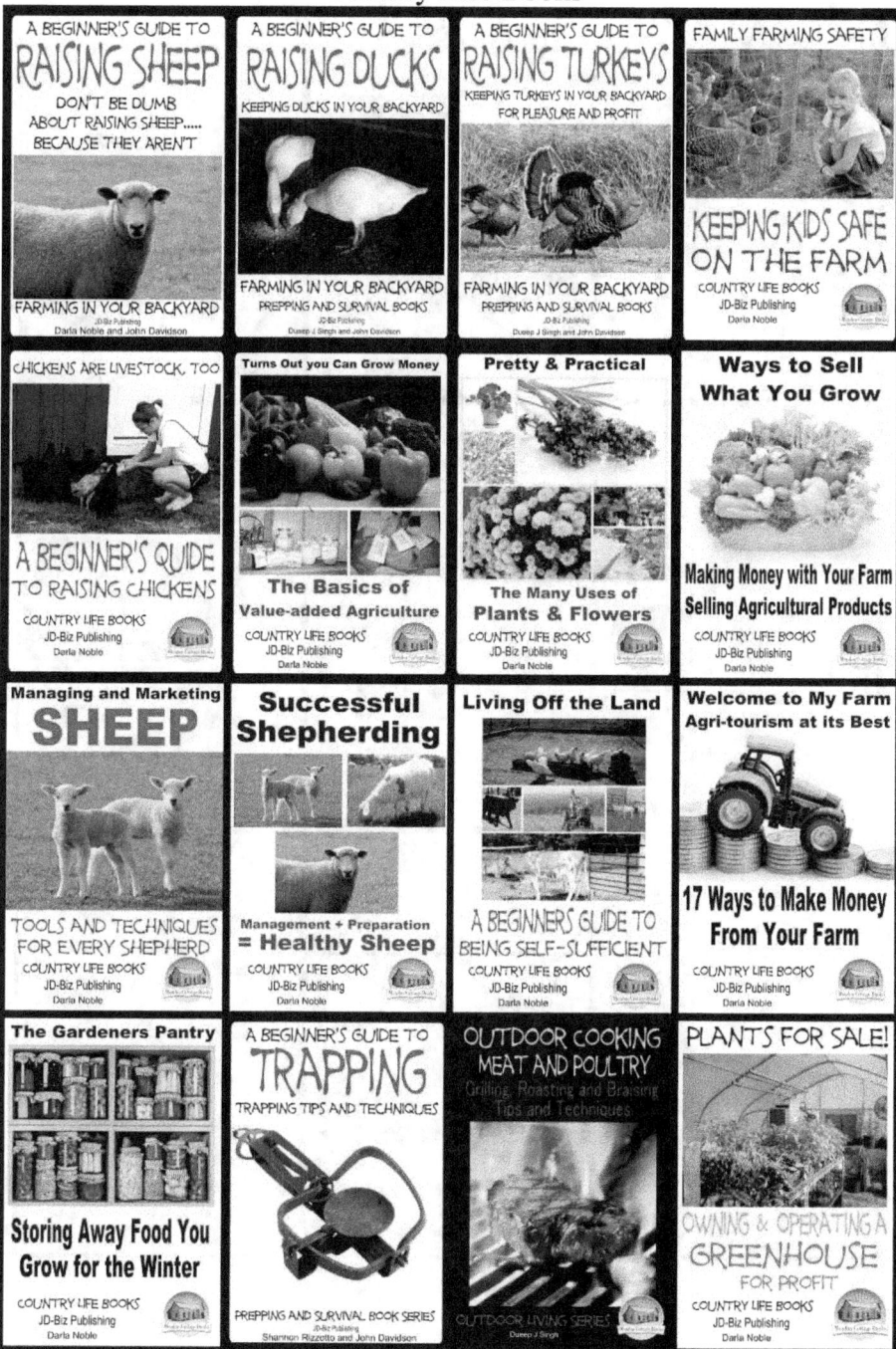

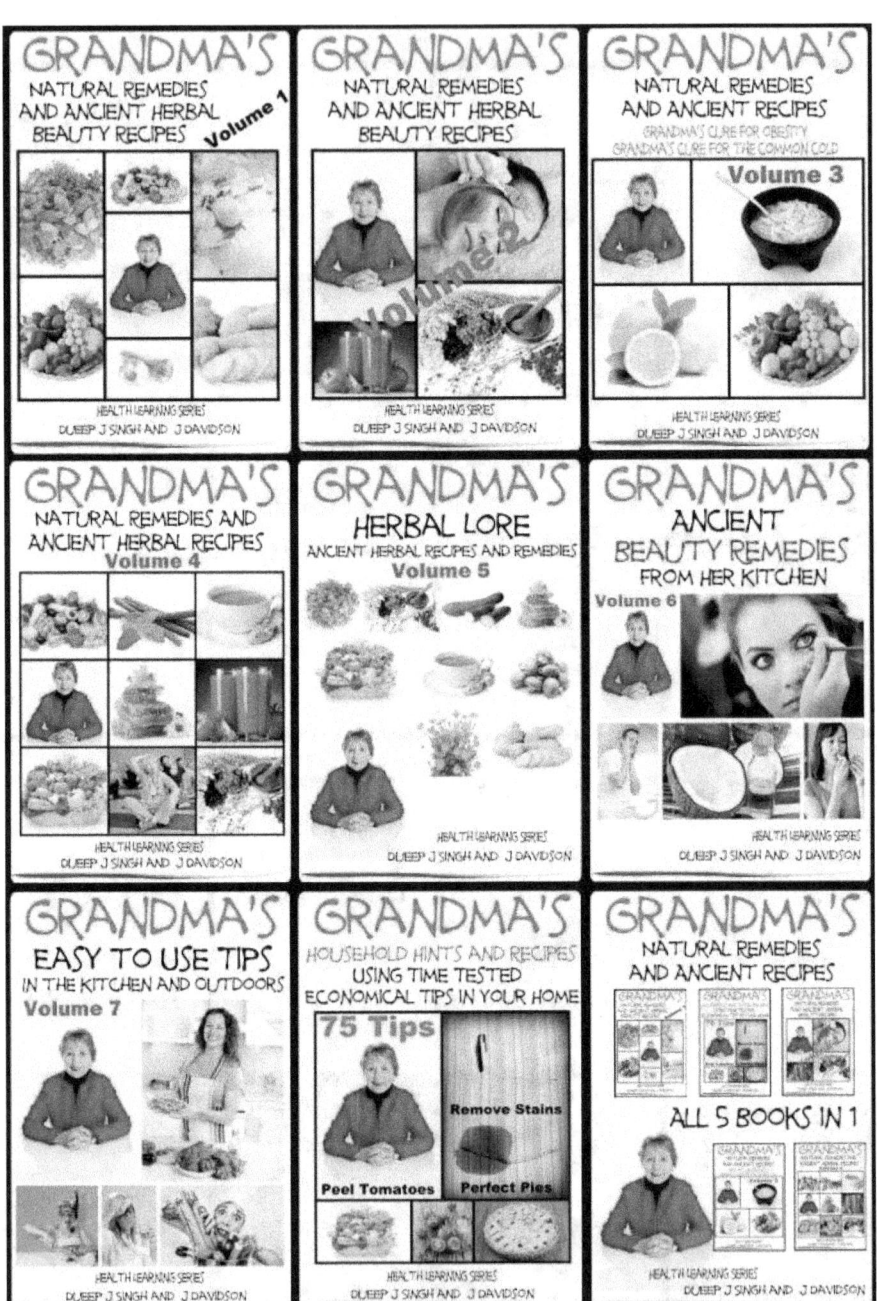

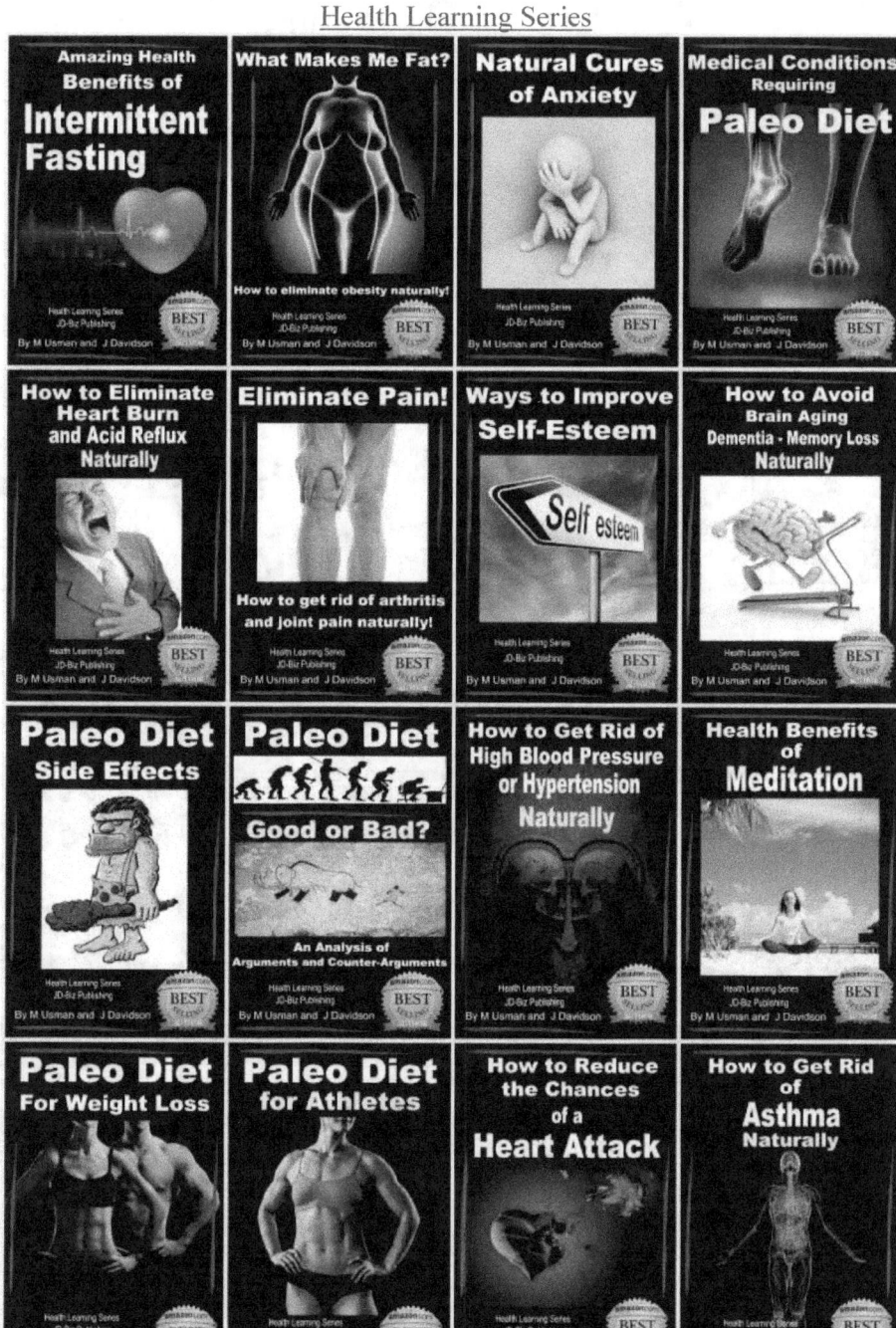

Amazing Animal Book Series

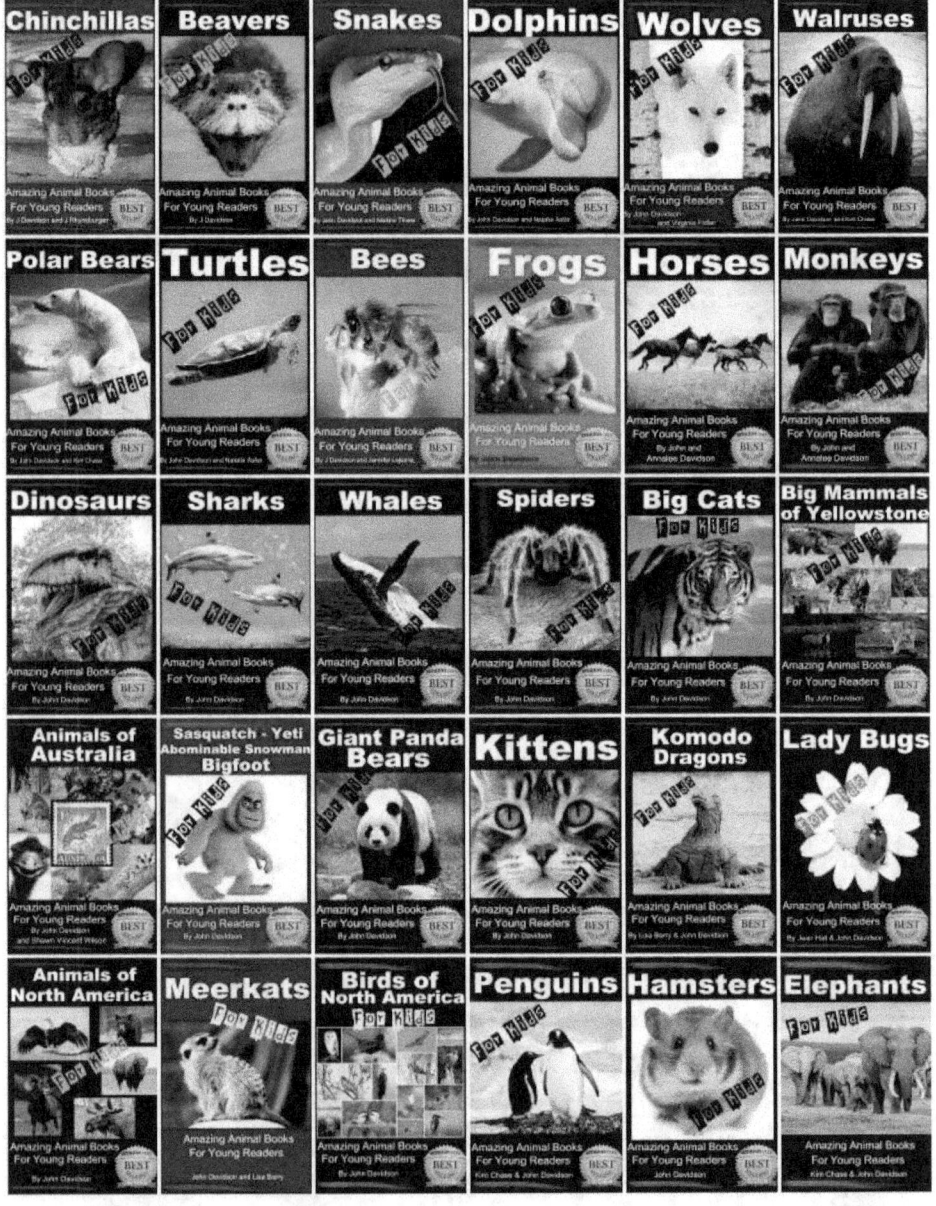

Learn To Draw Series

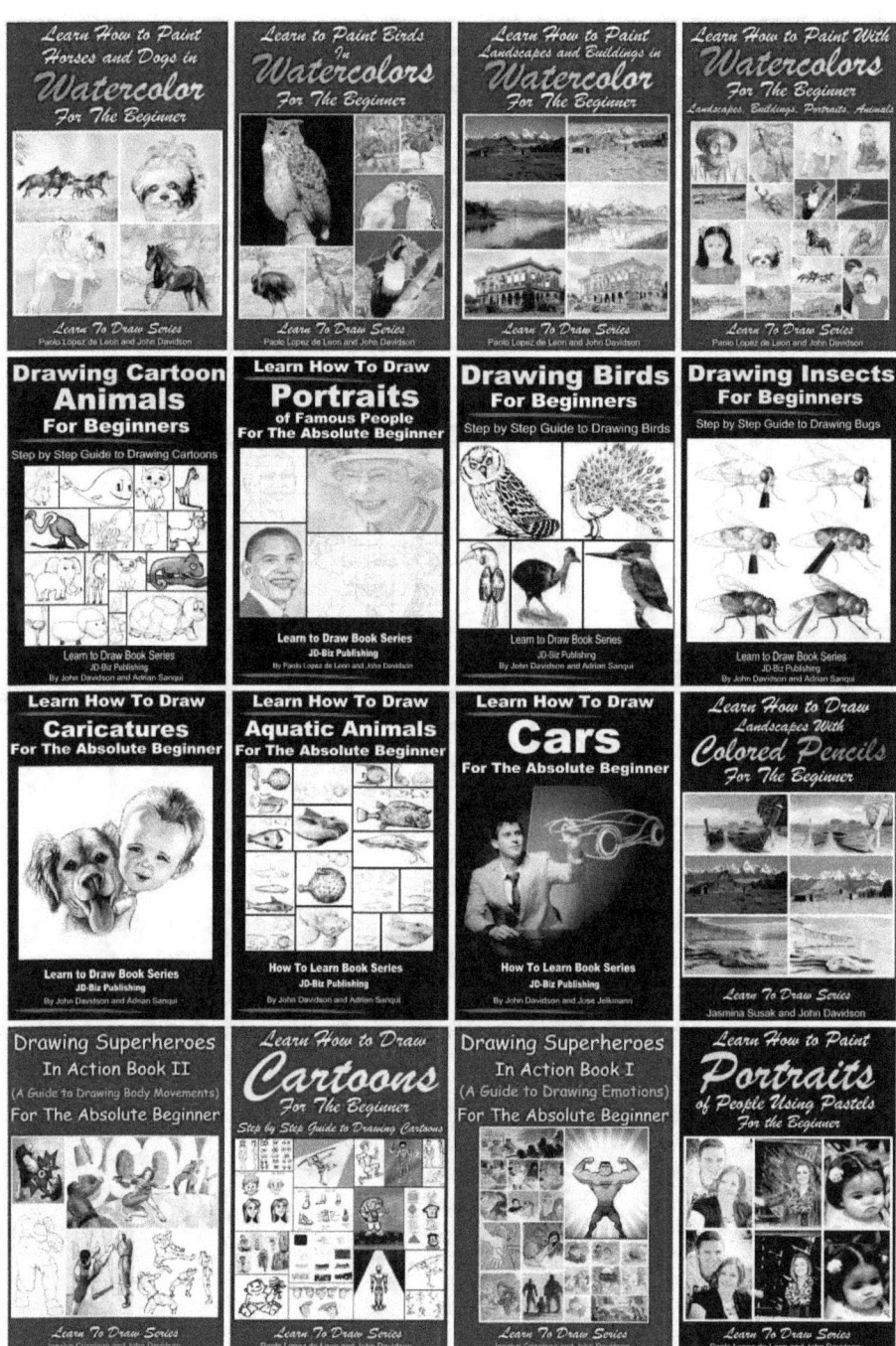

How to Build and Plan Books

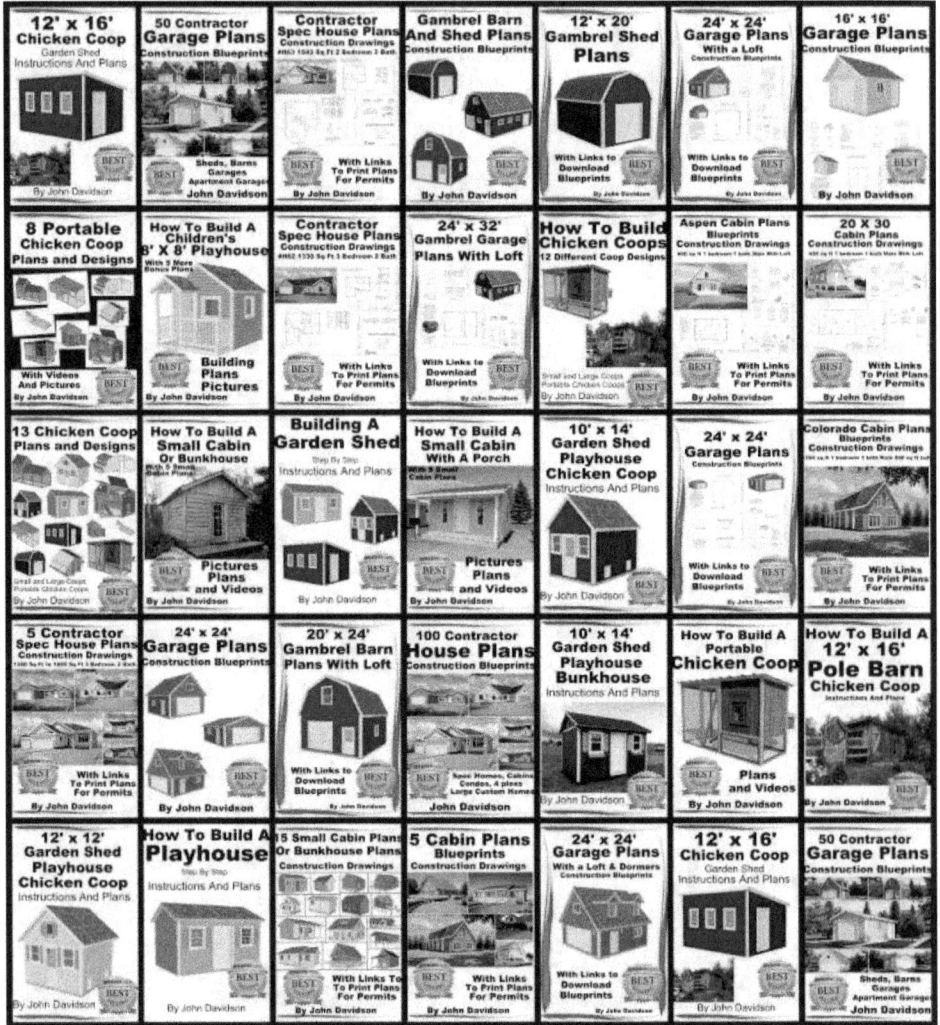

Entrepreneur Book Series

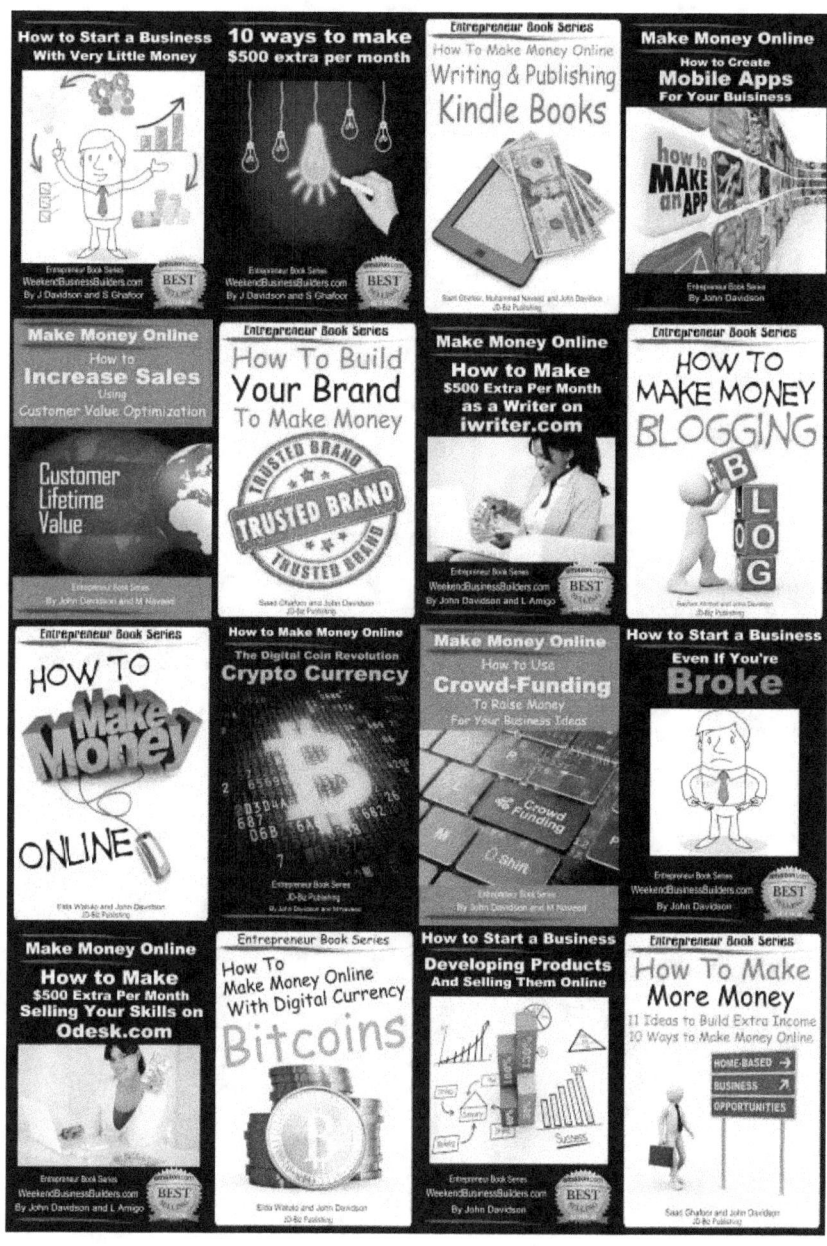

Our books are available at

1. Amazon.com

2. Barnes and Noble

3. Itunes

4. Kobo

5. Smashwords

6. Google Play Books

Download Free Books!

http://MendonCottageBooks.com

Publisher

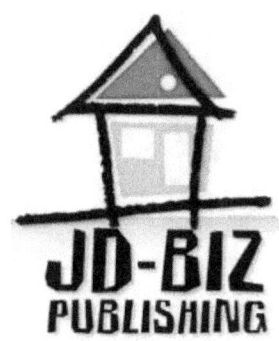

JD-Biz Corp

P O Box 374

Mendon, Utah 84325

http://www.jd-biz.com/

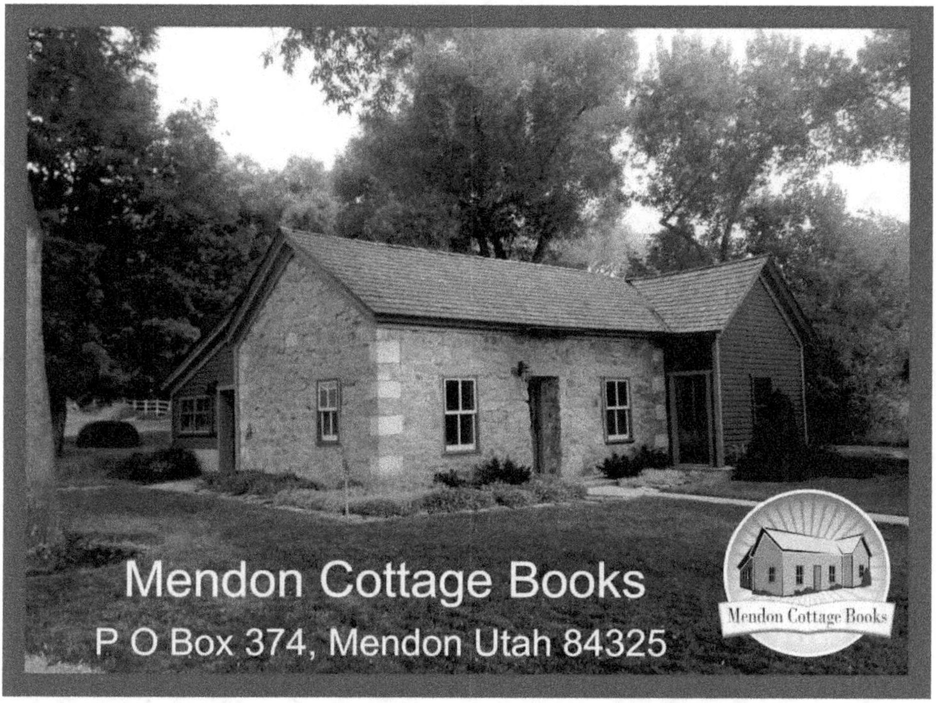

Mendon Cottage Books

P O Box 374, Mendon Utah 84325

Mendon Cottage Books